Hand sanitizer

Make your own homemade gel and spray to kill viruses and bacteria

By

Joe Romano

© Copyright 2020 by Joe Romano

All rights reserved.

This document is geared towards providing exact and reliable information with regard to the topic and issue covered. The publication is sold with the idea that the publisher is not required to render accounting, officially permitted, or otherwise qualified services. If advice is necessary, legal or professional, a practiced individual in the profession should be ordered.

From a Declaration of Principles which was accepted and approved equally by a Committee of the American Bar Association and a Committee of Publishers and Associations.

In no way is it legal to reproduce, duplicate, or transmit any part of this document in either electronic means or in printed format. Recording of this publication is strictly prohibited, and any storage of this document is not allowed unless with written permission from the publisher. All rights reserved.

The information provided herein is stated to be truthful and consistent, in that any liability, in terms of inattention or otherwise, by any usage or abuse of any policies, processes, or directions contained within is the solitary and utter responsibility of the recipient reader. Under no circumstances will any legal responsibility or blame be held against the publisher for any reparation, damages, or monetary loss due to the information herein, either directly or indirectly.

Respective authors own all copyrights not held by the publisher.

The information herein is offered for informational purposes solely and is universal as so. The presentation of the information is without a contract or any type of guarantee assurance.

The trademarks that are used are without any consent, and the publication of the trademark is without permission or backing by the trademark owner. All trademarks and brands within this book are for clarifying purposes only and are owned by the owners themselves, not affiliated with this document.

TABLE OF CONTENTS

INTRODUCTION

Hand sanitizer is a liquid or gel widely used on hands to reduce infectious agents. In most cases in the health care environment, alcohol-based style formulations are superior to handwashing with soap and water. It is generally more effective in destroying micro-organisms and is tolerated better than water and soap. Hand washing will also be performed if the damage can be noticed or after the toilet has been used. There are no guidelines for commonly using non-alcohol based models. Hand washing is generally preferred outside the health-care environment. Also, they are less successful for norovirus micro-organisms and Clostridium difficile. They come as oils, gels, and foams.

WHAT YOU SHOULD KNOW FIRST

The first thing to know is that, for at least 20 seconds, the best way to keep your hands clean is to wash them with soap and water. In addition to best practices when using a hand sanitizer, the Centers for Disease Control and Prevention (CDC) have hand washing instructions on their website. The CDC notes that while in some cases, "alcohol-based sanitizers will rapidly reduce the number of microbes on hands," they are not getting rid of any form of germ.

Furthermore, if you plan to make your hand sanitizer, note that you need to calculate the ingredients precisely for the product to function. Otherwise, you can do more harm than good.

Carl Fichtenbaum, an infectious disease specialist and clinical medicine professor at the University of Cincinnati, advises

Popular Mechanics that "It's not a bad idea" when it comes to DIY hand sanitizer. He also stresses the importance of product calculation for efficacy.

HOW TO USE HAND SANITIZER

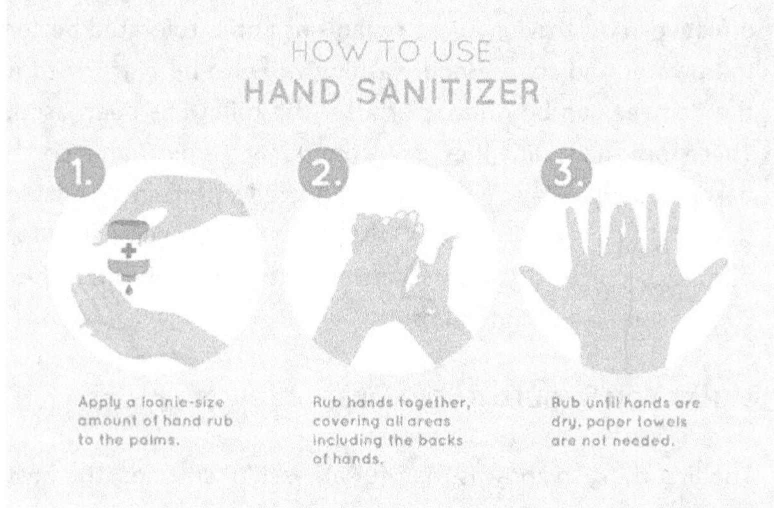

When using a hand sanitizer, two things to be mindful of are that you need to rub it into your skin before your hands are dry. And if your hands are greasy or dirty, you can first wash them with water and soap.

With that in mind, here are some tips for successful use of the hand sanitizer.

Spray the sanitizer or apply it to the palm of one hand.

Mix your palms vigorously together. Make sure you cover your hands and all your fingers all over the floor.

Continue to rub for 30-60 seconds or until the hands are dry. For hand sanitizer, it can take at least 60 seconds, and sometimes longer, to destroy most germs.

WHAT GERMS CAN DESTROY A SANITIZER BY HAND?

According to the CDCTrusted Source, a hand sanitizer based on alcohol that meets the requirement for the volume of alcohol will efficiently minimize the number of microbes on your hands. This can also help kill a wide variety of disease-causing agents or viruses on your hands, including the novel SARS-CoV coronavirus. However, even the best hand sanitizers based on alcohol have drawbacks and do not remove all forms of germs.

Hand sanitizers aren't going to get rid of potentially dangerous chemicals, according to the CDC. It is also not valid at destroying the following germs:

norovirus cryptosporidium (which causes cryptosporidiosis)

clostridiumdifficile (also known as C. diff)

And, if your hands are dirty or greasy, a hand sanitizer does not function well. This can happen after feeding, doing yard work, gardening, or playing a sport.

When your hands are dirty or slimy, instead of using a hand sanitizer, opt for handwashing.

Knowing when washing your hands is safe and when hand sanitizers may be beneficial is crucial to protecting yourself from the novel coronavirus and other diseases, such as common cold and seasonal flu.

While both serve a purpose, it should always be a priority to wash your hands with soap and water, according to the CDC. Using hand sanitizer only when you don't have soap and water in a given situation.

It's also necessary to always wash your hands. After going to the bathroom after blowing your nose, coughing, or sneezing before eating or touching infected surfaces, The CDC provides specific instructions Trusted Source on how to wash your hands most effectively. They suggest this: use warm, hot water at all times. (It can be hot or cold.) First, wash your hands, then shut off the shower, and later your hands with soap.

Clean your hands for at least 20 seconds with the soap. Make sure your hands are scrubbed between your fingers and under your nails.

Turn on the water and wash your face. Dry it using fresh air or a clean towel.

Benefits Of Hand Sanitizer

What are the benefits of using a hand sanitizer?

Hand sanitizers based on alcohol help to prevent the spread of germs and disease-causing bacteria, particularly in busy environments such as schools and offices: Stop the Spread of Germs: according to research, 1 in 5 people don't regularly wash their hands. Seventy percent of those who do, do not use soap. Providing hand sanitizer to kill harmful bacteria in critical areas (including bathrooms and kitchens) makes it more likely that people will be using it.

Promoting good hygiene and health: Successful construction is a safe house. An American Journal of Infection Control (AJIC) study found that promoting the use of hand sanitizers in schools decreased absenteeism by nearly 20%!

Reduce Waste: Most people will be using paper towels to open doors as they leave toilets or kitchens as an extra precaution. Placing hand sanitizers near exits makes it easy for humans to protect themselves against germs without creating an additional mess.

BENEFIT 1: CLEANLINESS This is not a surprise. One of hand sanitizer's main benefits is just that: it sanitizes. Such products have been designed to kill germs and do the job. Hand sanitizers will kill 99.9 percent of the bacteria on your hands when used correctly. The CDC suggests that you wash your hands whenever you are around food (preparing or consuming it), poultry, garbage, and more. When you find yourself in these circumstances, hand sanitizer is the perfect addition to washing your hands with soap and water (or sometimes substitute for it).

BENEFIT 2: PORTABILITY You cannot take a sink on the way the last time we checked. There isn't always going to be soap and water available in those cases where you need to wash your face. In your glove compartment, a purse, or even your wallet, you may slip a small bottle of hand sanitizer for circumstances where you might want to wash your hands but either you can't find a sink or it's inconvenient to wait for one (think long lines or far away from toilets). It's great for getting a snack at a sporting event or even leaving a public place, like the grocery store.

BENEFIT 3: Perfect FOR GROUP SETTINGS The germs spread rapidly at the workplace, in the classroom, or in any space with lots of foot traffic. And even if you're not getting ready to eat or take out the trash, you can be influenced (especially in close quarters) by the germs of others. For this reason, it is best for group settings to have hand sanitizer available. Teachers, teachers, and office staff may regularly destroy bacteria during the day without having to leave their classroom or desk, and gym-goers may use a hand sanitizer squirt before jumping on the next fitness machine.

BENEFIT 4: LESS RISK FOR DISEASE, Particularly during flu season, it is essential for your health to limit your exposure to other people's germs. You lower your risk of getting sick if you take a moment to sanitize your hands a few times during the day. Just a short trip to a friend's house or store will expose you to germs that could cause a cold, flu, or another disease, so it's essential to keep your hands as clean as possible.

BENEFIT 5: SOFTER-FEELING HANDS It may be one of hand sanitizer's most unexpected benefits, but it's not too good to be true. Hand sanitizers that do not contain alcohol will improve skin texture on your hands (note that alcohol-free hand sanitizers won't have this effect). Some hand sanitizers contain emollients softening your skin, giving your hands that look nicer and cleaner. You will undoubtedly notice a difference in the way your skin feels and looks moisturized. Avoid alcohol-containing hand sanitizers as they wash away the natural oils of the skin and can cause the skin to crack, which in turn creates an entry point for bacteria.

SHOULD WE AVOID HAND SANITIZERS?

1. DRY SKIN In a previous post, we told you about the dangers of alcohol in skincare. In hand sanitizers, the drinks used include isopropyl, ethanol, and n-propanol. These are the alcohols which we have told you about drying. They irritate the skin, extract natural oils and acid mantle, dehydrate cells, and increase the risk of dermatitis of touch.

2. ACCELERATED AGING All of these drying effects can lead to an improved appearance of fine lines and wrinkles, as well as calluses, cracks, and flakiness. Over time, alcohol can disrupt the role of the natural barrier, reduce the ability of the skin to defend itself, and lead to increased dehydration.

3. Scientific studies of DAMAGED SKIN have shown that alcohol can damage skin cells.

4. ANTIBIOTIC RESISTANCE These days, several hand sanitizers are made with triclosan (more on triclosan in this post). This antibacterial has been used for disrupting hormone activity in animal studies. It is also associated with the emergence of so-called "superbugs"— bacteria and viruses capable of avoiding antibiotics. In 2013, the CDC reported that the rise of superbugs (due to overuse of antibiotics) posed a significant threat to human health, causing at least 23,000 deaths that year.

5. UNKNOWN CHEMICALS There are many hand sanitizers made from chemical fragrances. Since manufacturers are not allowed to mention fragrance ingredients on the bottle, you are not aware of what you are exposed to. Most scents are

unpleasant and are associated with allergies and disturbance of the hormone.

6. WEAKENED IMMUNE SYSTEM We assume that when we use hand sanitizers, we reduce our chance of being sick. However, they can weaken the immune system. Studies have shown that ultra-clean environments— especially early in life — can later contribute to lowering immune defenses.

7. THEY JUST DON'T WORK AS WELL The FDA reports that there is currently no proof that antibacterial soaps (and sanitizers) are no more successful than regular soap and warm water to help prevent germ spread. A 2000 study found that sanitizers don't reduce the number of bacteria on the hands substantially, and can even increase it. Researchers added that the products strip the skin of its natural oils— and because those oils usually prevent bacteria from entering the surface, the sanitizer will also add to the skin's defenses.

WHERE SHOULD YOU PUT HAND SANITIZERS IN THE HOUSE?

You may think you have the cleanest hands in the world on Every Desk, but germs are crawling all over your desk. When you attach the bacteria to your computer mouse, keyboard, and phone, an average of 30,000 species would be present! Your best defense is a conventional sanitizer.

Through the Doors, Doorknobs are no secret to being hotbeds for bacteria. One germy handle could infect half the office within hours, according to CBS News! Your workers and guests are more likely to use a sanitizer at the entrance or exit if it is within reach of the head.

If Gary is in the middle of a compelling presentation in Meeting Rooms, spittle could be flying out of his mouth. Cold and flu viruses will live up to 18 hours on hard surfaces like the table in the boardroom! A few bottles of sanitizer can help avoid illness on your squad.

By the Elevator, after they cough into their mouth, eat a bag of Cheetos, or use the toilet, the colleagues touch their floor numbers or the arrows. It's no wonder that about 61 percent of elevator buttons are bacteria-contaminated. Do yourself a favor, and place a sanitizer on each floor on a tray.

Within the bathroom, it's unfortunately not always the case that the germs are gone when you leave the bathroom as lovely as it would be to believe. Currently, just 3 percent of people correctly wash their hands. A sanitizer is a good backup solution right outside the door, only in the event.

You may love the delicious sandwich in the kitchen or breakroom, but it contaminates your office kitchen or breakroom. Often filled with bacteria are the sink faucet, microwave handle, coffee maker, and refrigerator lid. Make sure that you use the sanitizer before and after consuming your meal.

How Is Hand Sanitizer Most Effectively Used?

It's essential to properly use hand sanitizer to ensure that it does the job it's meant to do—get rid of germs before they can spread: don't use hand sanitizer if your hands are dirty: hand sanitizers are not intended to clean your hands. Disinfecting contaminants such as oil or soil can prevent hand sanitizers from touching the skin.

Using the Right Amount: The less does not equal more when it comes to hand sanitizer. You must add enough to cover every part of your hands thoroughly. Don't think about their back or your hand!

Rub It In Before Your Hands Are Dry: This way, you can be sure that all the most essential surfaces come into contact with it.

Combined with other prevention steps (such as regular hand washing and thorough touch-point cleaning), the use of a hand sanitizer can help to protect you (and everyone in your building!) from the flu and other diseases.

Hand Sanitizer vs. Handwashing: Which Is Best for Preventing the Spread of Germs?

Hands are the areas of our body that have the most interaction with other people, things, and our selves — think of how much you mindlessly touch your face during the day. And while head-to-toe hygiene is a high priority for so many people, there is also a robust emphasis on keeping the hands clean when it comes to preventing disease-carrying germs from spreading.

If you've always been hands-on sanitizer or prefer soap and water cleaning, you're still ahead of the game. In essence, both are much better at reducing the spread of certain viruses and bacteria than doing anything to purify your hands. Yet does one solution work better than the other? To get to the bottom of which approach is best for holding germs at bay, we consulted with medical experts.

Hand sanitizer Hand sanitizer's pros and cons have become a staple of purses, bags, and on keychains— and with good reason. "Hand sanitizer can be more compact and available while people are on the go, which will increase the number of times they will wash their hands. It will also minimize the risk of viruses being spread," says Neha Nanda, University of Southern California's medical director of infection prevention and anti-microbial stewardship at Keck Medicine.

Niket Sonpal, an internist, gastroenterologist, and adjunct professor at Touro College in New York, agrees that it may sometimes be the most convenient option: "The benefit of a hand sanitizer is the opportunity to combat germs when water and soap are not immediately available." Sonpal adds that hand sanitizers are efficient in neutralizing specific pathogens, viruses, and bacteria— but not everything.

"Hand sanitizers are active against all forms of viruses except norovirus, which causes some form of diarrhea," explains Linda Anegawa, an internist with PlushCare based in Hawaii. They are, therefore, not a complete prophylactic though indeed serving a useful function. "Sanitizers often don't protect against other forms of bacteria, including one named C. difficile, which causes antibiotic overuse diarrhea." AthanasiosMelisiotis, a Penn Medicine physician at the University of Pennsylvania, points out some other possible hand sanitizer downsides: "Some hand sanitizers can leave a residue that some consumers feel sticky or unpleasant," he says. "Hand sanitizers are nice in a pinch and are more convenient, but ultimately soap and water are better." Why doctors prefer soap and water, and why many homes and businesses have large pump bottles of hand sanitizers readily available, it's safer to use hand sanitizer as a compact option when a sink and soap are not accessible. Why? For what? "Viruses are most easily destroyed even with soap and water separated from the mouth," Nanda says.

"The consensus between CDC and medical practitioners alike is that proper and regular hand washing is the gold standard for preserving hand hygiene," Sonpal tells Allure. That's because the water and soap are even more detailed.

"Hand sanitizer can destroy viruses and other bacteria, but as soap and water do, it does not' clean' your hands," Melisiotis says. "Sanitizer doesn't absorb dirt and particles. Soap removes germs, separates them, and helps physically clean them, water, skin, and drain." This might sound that using an antibacterial soap will be the best in all worlds, and although it's not a terrible thing, the jury is still out about whether or not it's better than standard soap. "Some soaps are enough. If you want to go the extra mile with antibacterial soaps you can, but CDC tests have shown that using antibacterial soap over normal soap has little added value," Sonpal says.

When soap and water are not available, what to look for in a hand sanitizer if your only choice is hand sanitizer, make sure that the one you're carrying is really up to scratch, which means the ingredients test. "If water and soap are not available immediately, hand sanitizers with up to 60 percent alcohol are fine second alternatives," says Sonpal. Anegawa agrees, adding that customers are searching for up to 95 percent ethanol or isopropanol through the FDA.

"Ignore 'drug-free' sanitizers because there is not enough evidence on them, and they can differ in efficacy. We know that alcohol destroys viruses," says Melisiotis. "Nevertheless, do not make your hand sanitizer. You can purchase quality-controlled and tested products that have efficient sanitation." Michael Chang, a UTHealth infectious disease specialist at the University of Texas in Houston, says there are several hand sanitizers with a benzalkonium chloride ingredient that has been shown to kill bacteria and viruses but not as much as alc. "Ironically, benzalkonium chloride is active against norovirus, but for most respiratory viruses, such as seasonal flu or this recent [COVID-19 coronavirus], it is preferred to use alcohol-based hand sanitizers." Another justification for sticking to alcohol-based hand sanitizers: "Because the alcohol in the sanitizer acts as a preservative, it is less likely to be infected than alcohol-free sanitizers."

Anegawa warns even against the introduction of another common ingredient: triclosan. She says it's believed this specific antibacterial agent may decrease a hand sanitizer's efficacy and may also lead to bacterial resistance.

Anything you use, the procedure is essential. If you're using soap and water or a hand sanitizer, if you don't use the right techniques, you may as well be using nothing. "The type of soap used is less important than the way you wash your hands," Nanda says. Each professional we spoke to insisted on scrubbing for at least 20 seconds with soap and water — Chang also insists on a minimum of 40 seconds— so a splash of soap on the palms followed by an almost immediate rinse won't cut it.

And you may be shocked to hear that the guidelines are much stricter for proper hand sanitizer use. "The CDC cites a three-step method: liberally apply the sanitizer, rub palms together to cover all surfaces, and rub until the hands are fully dry," explains Anegawa. The WHO Guidelines build upon the second step of the CDC, clarifying that users of hand sanitizers should rub their right palm over the back of their left hand with interlaced fingers (and vice versa), rub palm to palm with interlaced fingers, and rub their finger back to opposing palms with interlaced fingers.

"Sanitizers based on alcohol work by breaking down the germs, so you don't just need to have enough, the alcohol needs to stick around long enough to work," Chang says, advising that you rub your hands with a sanitizer until they're entirely air-dry. "That usually ensures adequate exposure time. The exposure time always needs to be more than 20 seconds. If you're only pumping adequate sanitizer to make your hands dry in 5 to 10 seconds, it's probably not enough." But in the end, Chang says, it's down to doing it. "In the end, I generally suggest whatever you are most likely to do the most often, regularly, and correctly would be the most successful way to avoid the spread of infection," he recommends. "Otherwise, why not do both?"

WORLD HEALTH ORGANIZATION RECIPE FOR HOMEMADE HAND SANITIZER

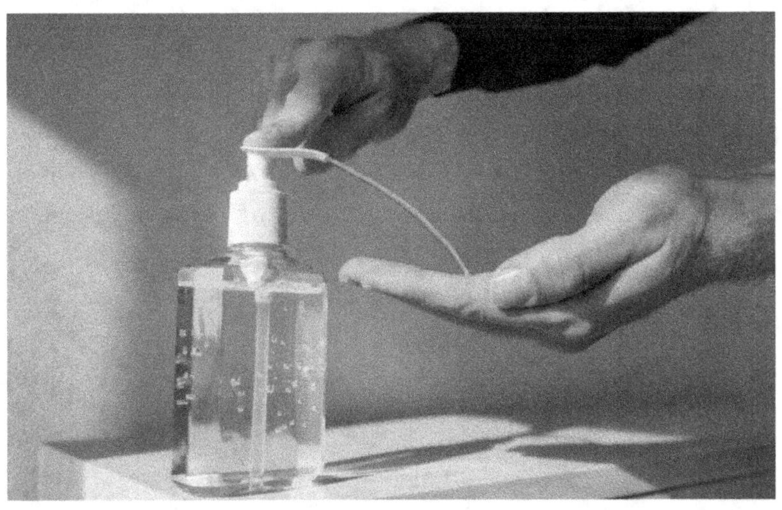

WHO's DIY hand sanitizer recipe can seem like a last-ditch effort, and while many of the ingredients required to produce the formulations at home can sound unusual, they can be bought online or at a local pharmacy.

"A WHO expert group's consensus is that hand rub formulation recommended by the WHO may be used for both hygienic hand antiseptic and presurgical hand preparation," the WHO reported.

If one is not available, the WHO has given two separate formulas in their alcohol bases.

Such alcohol-based hand rubs, according to WHO, are a known means of quickly and efficiently inactivating a wide variety of potentially harmful micro-organisms on palms. The

Centers for Disease Control and Prevention suggests using at least 60 percent alcohol with a hand sanitizer.

Here's what you need to make your hand sanitizer, according to WHO:

- 8333 ml (2.2 gallons) of 96% ethanol or 7515 ml (2 gallons) of 99.8% isopropyl alcohol
- 417 ml (1.76 cups G) of 3% hydrogen peroxide, which is used to inactivate contaminating bacterial spores in the solution and it's not an active agent for hand antisepsis
- 145 ml of 98% glycerol
- Wooden, plastic or metal mixing paddles
- Measuring tubes and weighing jugs
- Plastic or metal funnel

The organization's formula can be prepared in 10-liter glass or plastic bottles with screw-threaded stoppers to prevent spillage.

According to WHO, here is the step-by-step preparation: The alcohol for the solution to be used is poured into the large bottle or tank to the graduated point.

The hydrogen peroxide is added using the measuring cylinder.

Glycerol is applied through a cylinder for calculation. Since glycerol is very viscous and sticks to the wall of the measuring container, some sterile distilled or cold boiled water should be rinsed and then poured into the bottle/tank.

The bottle/tank is then filled with sterile distilled or cold boiled water up to the 10-liter limit.

After preparation, the lid of the screw cap is mounted on the tank/bottle as soon as possible, to avoid evaporation.

The solution is combined by shaking gently or using a paddle, where necessary.

Place the solution into quarantine 72 hours before use. This gives time for the removal of any spores found in the alcohol or the new / re-used bottles.

The World Health Organization has released a guide to producing large amounts of chemical hand sanitizers available in developing countries where commercial hand sanitizers might not be available. According to this guide, the following are blended to create 10 liters of hand sanitizer and topped with distilled or cold boiled water to 10 liters:

- 8333 ml of 96% ethanol, 417 ml of 3% hydrogen peroxide, and 145 ml of 98% glycerol, or
- 7515 ml of 99.8% isopropyl alcohol, 417 ml of 3% hydrogen peroxide, and 145 ml of 98% glycerol.

Such proportions equate to 0.8333x96=80 percent ethanol or 0.7515x99.8= 75 percent isopropyl alcohol, thus meeting the 60 percent as mentioned above to 95 percent volume concentration range. A more straightforward solution for individuals is to add ~15 ml of glycerin or aloe vera gel to 1 L of ~90 percent denatured alcohol or rubbing alcohol plus, as a general disinfectant, ultimately 40 ml of 3 percent hydrogen peroxide. This composition will also reach the appropriate range of alcohol concentration, without the need to add water. All this and the WHO formulations are less viscous than industrial sanitizer spray, and they are a more significant fire threat, like alcohol.

Types of Automatic hand sanitizer Alcohol-based hand rubs are commonly used as an alternative to antiseptic soaps in the hospital environment. Hand-rubs have two uses in the hospital environment: hygienic cleaning of hands and surgical hand disinfection. Hand rubs based on alcohol have more excellent resistance to the skin compared with antiseptic soap. Hand rubs also show more powerful microbiological properties than antiseptic soaps in contrast.

Often used in hospital hand-rubs are the same ingredients used in over-the-counter hand rubs: alcohols such as ethanol and isopropanol, often mixed with quaternary ammonium cations (quats) such as benzalkonium chloride. Quats are applied at rates up to 200 parts per million to improve the potency of anti-microbials. Although allergy to alcohol-only rubs is uncommon, fragrances, preservatives, and quats can trigger allergies to the touch. Such other additives do not evaporate like alcohol and remain until they are drained with soap and water, leaving a "sticky" residue.

The most popular brands of hand rubbing alcohol include Aniosgel, Avant, Sterillium, Desderman, and Allsept S. All hand rubs in hospitals must comply with specific regulations, such as EN 12054 for hand-rubbing hygienic care and surgical disinfection. In the hospital environment, goods with a claim of "99.99 percent reduction" or 4-log reduction are unsuccessful, as the modification must be more than "99.99 percent."

The hospital-based hand sanitizer dosing systems are designed to provide a measured amount of the drug to workers. They are dosing pumps that are mounted onto a bottle or are dispensers with refill bottles explicitly designed. Containers for surgical hand disinfection are typically fitted with an elbow-controlled mechanism or infrared sensors to prevent any interaction with the device.

Surgical hand disinfection Hands have to be disinfected by hand washing with mild soap and then hand-rubbing with a sanitizer before any surgical operation. Surgical disinfection requires a higher hand-rub dosage, and a longer rubbing time than average. It is generally performed in two procedures using different hand-rubbing methods, EN1499 (hygienic hand wash) and EN 1500 (hygienic hand disinfection), to ensure that antiseptic is added to the surface of the hand everywhere.

ALCOHOL-BASED HAND SANITIZER

Usually, alcohol-based formulations contain a mixture of isopropyl alcohol, ethanol (ethyl alcohol), or n-propanol. The most potent forms are containing 60 to 95 percent alcohol. Care should be taken because it is flame-retardant. Hand sanitizer dependent on alcohol acts against several micro-organisms but not spores. Other products contain compounds such as glycerol to prevent skin from drying. Non-alcohol based versions can contain triclosan or benzalkonium chloride.

Alcohol was used at least as early as 1363 as an antiseptic, with evidence to support its use becoming available in the late 1800s. Manual hand sanitizer based on alcohol has been widely used in Europe since at least the 1980s. The alcohol-based version is on the list of essential drugs, the safest and most effective medicines needed in a health system, issued by the World Health Organisation. In the developing world, the wholesale cost is about US$ 1.40–3.70 per liter bottle.

Using The U.S. Centers for Disease Control and Prevention (CDC)'s Safe Hands program instructs the public to wash hands. Hand sanitizer based on alcohol is only recommended in the absence of soap and water.

When using a hand sanitizer based on alcohol: Apply the drug to the palm of one hand.

Rub your face.

Apply the drug on both hand and finger surfaces until the hands are washed.

The latest evidence for hand hygiene measures in schools is of low quality.

Health care Hand alcohol in a hospital An automatic hand sanitizer dispenser hand sanitizer Alcohol-based hand sanitizer is more convenient than handwashing with soap and water in most health-care cases. It is usually more effective in destroying micro-organisms and tolerated better than soap and water. Hand washing can always be done where waste can be observed or after the toilet is used.

Hand sanitizer should be used, which contains at least 60 percent alcohol or a "persistent antiseptic." Alcohol rubs destroy several different types of bacteria, including bacteria that are resistant to antibiotics and bacteria that have TB. 90% Alcohol rubber is extremely flammable but destroys many forms of viruses, including enveloped viruses such as flu virus, common cold virus, coronavirus, and HIV. However, it is especially ineffective against rabies.

Alcohol rubs are 90 percent more effective against viruses than most other types of handwashing. For less than 30 seconds, both in the laboratory and on human skin, isopropyl alcohol can kill 99.99 percent or more of all non-spore forming bacteria.

For hand sanitizers, alcohol does not have the exposure time of 10–15 seconds needed to denature proteins and lysis cells is too small (0.3 ml) or concentrations (less than 60 percent). In conditions with high lipids or protein waste (such as food processing), it may not be necessary to use alcohol hand rubs alone to ensure proper hand hygiene.

In health care environments such as hospitals and clinics, the optimal concentration of alcohol to kill bacteria is between 70% and 95%. According to researchers at East Tennessee State University, items with alcohol concentrations as low as 40 percent are available in American stores.

Sanitizers to rub alcohol destroy most bacteria and fungi, and avoid some viruses. Chemical rubbing sanitizers that contain at least 70% chemical (mainly ethyl alcohol) kill 99.9% of the bacteria in hands 30 seconds after application and 99.99% to 99.99% in one minute.

For health care, optimal disinfection needs attention to all visible surfaces, including under the fingernails, between the fingertips, on the back of the thumb, and around the hand. For a time of at least 30 seconds, hand alcohol should be thoroughly rubbed into the hands and on the lower forearm, then allowed to air dry.

The use of alcohol-based hand gels dries skinless, leaving more moisture in the epidermis than antiseptic /anti-microbial soap and water washing with hands.

Drawbacks certain conditions in which handwashing with water and soap is favored over hand sanitizer to include:

Removal of Clostridioidesdifficile bacterial spores, parasites such as Cryptosporidium, and other viruses such as norovirus, depending on the concentration of alcohol in the sanitizer (95 percent of alcohol was found to be most efficient in removing certain infections). However, if hands are contaminated with fluids or other visible pollutants, hand washing is recommended both after usage of the toilet and if irritation occurs from the result of the use of the alcohol sanitizer.[36]

CDC reports hand sanitizers are not effective in eliminating chemicals such as pesticides.

Security Fire Alcohol gel will catch fire, which creates a transparent blue flame. That is because the gel contains flammable alcohol. Some hand sanitizer gels due to a high concentration of water or moisturizing agents do not produce this effect. There have been several unusual cases where alcohol was involved in causing fires in the operating room, including a case where alcohol used as an antiseptic collected in an operating room under the surgical drapes and sparked a fire while using a cautery tool. Alcohol gel was not involved.

Alcohol rub users are advised to rub their hands until dry, which means that the flammable alcohol has evaporated, to mitigate the risk of fire. Fire departments recommend that refills for alcohol-based hand sanitizers should be kept away from heat sources or open flames with cleaning supplies.

Skin Research indicates that by removing beneficial micro-organisms that are naturally present on the skin, alcohol hand sanitizers pose little risk. The body replenishes the beneficial microbes on the hands rapidly, often bringing them in from just up the arms where less dangerous micro-organisms are present.

Alcohol may strip the skin of the outer layer of oil, however, which can have adverse effects on the skin's barrier function. Research also indicates that disinfecting hands with an anti-microbial detergent contributes to a more significant destruction of skin barriers compared to alcohol solutions, indicating an increased loss of skin lipids.

Intake In the United Kingdom, the United Nations Food and Drug Administration (FDA) regulates hand-held anti-microbial soaps and sanitizers as over-the-counter drugs (OTCs) since they are intended for topical anti-microbial use to avoid human disease. The FDA requires strict labeling to inform consumers of the proper use of this OTC drug and to avoid hazards, including warning adults not to ingest, not to use in the eyes, to keep children out of reach, and to allow children to use it only under adult supervision. There were almost 12,000 cases of hand sanitizer ingestion in 2006, according to the American Association of Poison Control Centers. When swallowed, hand sanitizers based on alcohol can cause alcohol poisoning in infants. Yet the U.S. Centers for Disease Control recommends using hand sanitizer for children to encourage good health, under supervision, and also supports parents packing hand sanitizer for their children while traveling, to prevent their dirty hands catching the illness.

Incidents of people consuming the gel have been recorded in prisons and hospitals where alcohol intake is not allowed to become intoxicated, leading to its removal from some establishments.

Non-Alcohol Based

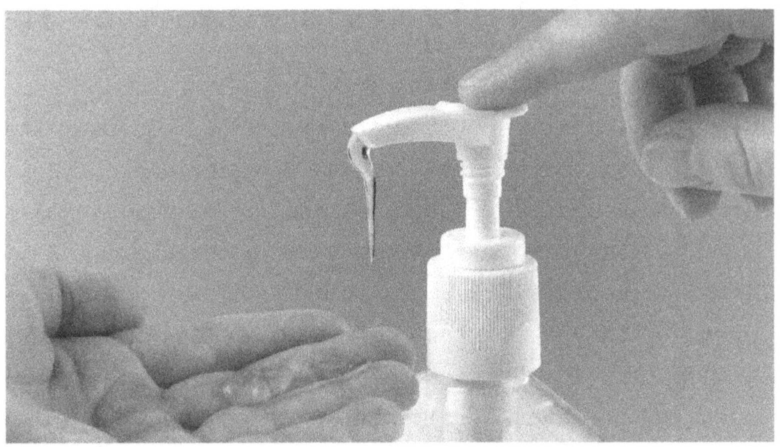

Many hand sanitizer products use chemicals other than alcohol to destroy micro-organisms, such as povidone-iodine, benzalkonium chloride, or triclosan.

The World Health Organization (WHO) and the CDC suggest hand sanitizers with "persistent" antiseptics. Persistent activity is described as the prolonged or extended anti-microbial activity, which, after application of the product, prevents or inhibits the proliferation or survival of micro-organisms. This behavior can be demonstrated by sampling a site several minutes or hours after use and showing the efficacy of bacterial anti-microbials relative to a baseline point. This property has often been referred to as "residual infection." Both substantive and non-substantive active ingredients will display a persistent effect if the number of bacteria during the wash cycle is significantly reduced.

Laboratory experiments have been shown to link residual benzalkonium chloride with antibiotic resistance in MRSA.

Alcohol sanitizers can build tolerance in fecal bacteria. Where alcohol sanitizers use 62%, or higher, by weight alcohol, just 0.1 to 0.13% by weight of benzalkonium chloride has equal anti-microbial efficacy.

Triclosan has been shown to accumulate in biosolids in the atmosphere, one of the top seven organic pollutants in wastewater under the National Toxicology Program Triclosan leads to numerous issues with natural biological systems, and triclosan produces dioxins, a possible carcinogen in humans. However, 90–98 percent of triclosan in wastewater biodegrades by both photolytic and natural biological processes or is eliminated in wastewater treatment plants due to sorption. Numerous experiments indicate that only microscopic traces in the effluent water entering the rivers are observable.

Several studies show that triclosanphotodegradation produced 2,4-dichlorophenol and 2,8-dichlorodibenzo-p-dioxin (2,8-DCDD). The 2,4-dichlorophenol itself is considered to be both biodegradable and photodegradable. A conversion rate of 1 percent has been recorded for DCDD, one of the dioxin family's non-toxic compounds, and approximate half-lives indicate it is also photolabile. DCDD's formation-decay kinetics are also stated by Sanchez-Prado et al. (2006), who says that "triclosan transformation to toxic dioxins has never been demonstrated and is highly unlikely." Alcohol-free hand sanitizers may be successful immediately when on the skin. Still, the solutions themselves can become contaminated because alcohol is an in-solution preservative, and without it, the alcohol-from-skin. However, even alcohol-containing hand sanitizers can become infected if the alcohol content is not adequately monitored or the sanitizer during manufacture is heavily contaminated with micro-organisms. In June 2009, the FDA removed alcohol-free Clarion Antimicrobial Hand Sanitizer from the US market, which found that the drug contained exceptionally high levels of contamination of various bacteria, including those that could "cause opportunistic skin and underlying tissue infections and could result in medical or surgical treatment and permanent damage." Gross contamination of any hand sanitizer by bacteria during fabrication would fail the sanitizer's effectiveness and potential infection of the treatment site with the contaminating organisms.

On 30 April 2015, the FDA announced it was seeking more scientific evidence focused on hand sanitizer health. Emerging research also indicates that systemic exposure (full body exposure as shown by identification of antiseptic ingredients in the blood or urine) is higher than previously thought for at least some health care antiseptic active ingredients, and current evidence poses potential concerns about the conscquences of prolonged everyday human exposure to certain antiseptic active ingredients. That would include alcohol-and triclosan-containing hand sterile products.

Composition Hand sanitizers focused on alcohol and health care "mouth alcohol" or "chemical mouth antiseptic agents" are available in formulations of liquid, foam, and easy-to-flow gel. Goods containing alcohol by volume from 60 to 95 percent are potent antiseptics. Lower or higher concentrations are less effective; the majority of products contain alcohol between 60 and 80 percent.

In addition to alcohol (ethanol, isopropanol or n-Propanol), hand sanitizers often include the following: additional antiseptics such as chlorhexidine and quaternary ammonium derivatives, sporicides such as hydrogen peroxides that remove bacterial spores which may be present in ingredients, emollients and gelling agents to minimize dryness and inflammation of the skin, a small amount of sterile.

3 Laws of Hand Sanitizers

By now, everyone should be aware that a hand sanitizer is essential to preserving health and protecting the immune system from germs. The Centers for Disease Control (CDC) has told us that in addition to regular and thorough washing of your hands, using a hand sanitizer to remove germs is highly effective in minimizing the risk of colds and cases of flu, among other diseases. Below are the three laws to search for when a strong hand sanitizer is being sought.

The Law of Effectiveness You need a hand sanitizer that WORKS to be viable as a sanitizing product. Several drugs are on the market, but the FDA expressly licensed those substances as anti-microbials. And ethyl, alcohol is one of those compounds. Ethyl alcohol can be effective against germs at 99.9 percent in the right quantities. The typical sum by volume is about 62-70 percent. If a hand sanitizer does not contain a drug approved by the FDA, such as ethyl alcohol, you can't be sure it is safe.

Sanitizing the Rule of Application Hand isn't something that most people do daily. The issue is they should be, but the majority of hand sanitizers are a pain to be applied. You have to take out a small teenage bottle, open the cap, squeeze out the gel in the right quantity and try to spread it on your hands until it slips off or evaporates. It is an easy feat for those with more than two hands, but it's a bit difficult for the rest of us. The best application for hand sanitizer is via a spray bottle, which gives you the right amount per spray and is very easy to do with two hands. If the hand sanitizer can't be quickly applied, why should you be able to use it?

The Law on Moisture Alcohol is a solvent that removes natural oils, like your skin, from anything it touches. This dries out as the skin loses its natural oils. This can be painful, and perhaps why people don't want to use hand sanitizers ANOTHER explanation. That's why the Moisture Law says you have a hand sanitizer with aloe or some kind of essential oils! After you rub it around to destroy germs, the alcohol will evaporate, and then you will be left with an excellent moisturizing solution that will protect your hands from getting bruised and sore.

Follow these laws to find a decent hand-sanitizing product that isn't going to be a pain to use! Hand sanitizing is one of the easiest ways to stop being sick, so don't be afraid anymore-follow the three-hand sanitizer laws and protect yourself!

Jodi M. Smith. She is a mom who is passionate about keeping her family safe. She strongly suggests using a systematic program strategy to protect against cold and flu. Her favorite drug is a hand sanitizer spray for ultimate prevention. Use a shower instead of a gel aids in absorption and makes it easier for children to apply. Because we all know children need more than anyone to fight bacteria! To aloe and acai added value, your hands will never feel better! As part of a full line of cold and flu items, Sun Dew allows a clinically formulated hand sanitizer to help protect, encourage, improve, and treat you and your family 365 days a year.

TWO EASY HOMEMADE RECIPES

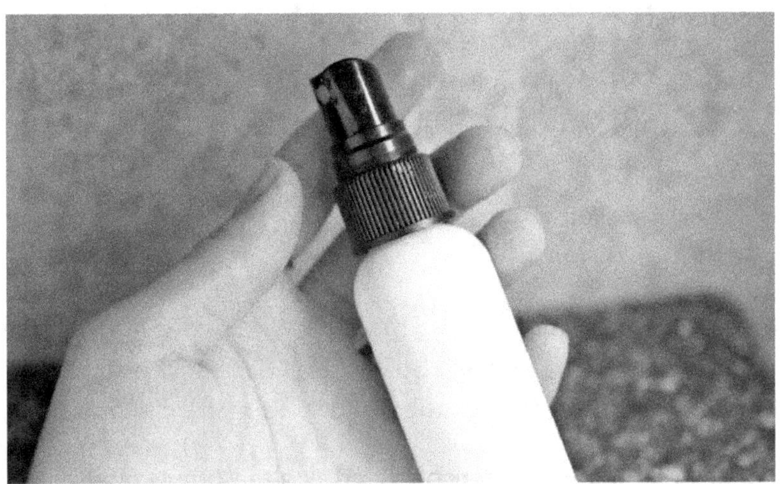

THE FAST (GEL) RECIPE

Ingredients:

- Isopropyl Alcohol
- Aloe Vera Gel
- Tea Tree Oil

Mix 3 parts of alcohol isopropyl to 1 part aloe vera. To give it a pleasant fragrance, and align your chakras, add a few drops of tea tree oil.

THE BEST (SPRAY) RECIPE

Ingredients:

- Isopropyl alcohol
- Glycerol or Hydrogen peroxide
- Glycerin
- Distilled water
- Spray bottle

The aloe combination does the job, but aloe leaves the skin annoyingly sticky as well. So, here's a less sticky and more potent formula, based on the blend WHO recommends.

Mix 12 fluid ounces of alcohol and two teaspoons of glycerol. You can buy glycerol jugs online, and this is a vital ingredient as it prevents the alcohol from drying your hands out. When you can't find glycerol, go ahead with the rest of the recipe and just try to moisturize your hands after the sanitizer is applied.

Add in 1 teaspoon of hydrogen peroxide, then three distilled or boiled (and cooled) fluid ounces of water. (If you deal with a lower alcohol concentration solution, use even less water; note, alcohol must be at least 3/4 of the final mix.) Load the solution into spray bottles— this is not a solvent; it is a spray. Using it, you can even wet a paper towel and use it as a wipe.

Will Vodka Work? What You Need to Know About Using Hand Sanitizers Against Coronavirus

1. How is alcohol the most active ingredient in the hand sanitizers?

Alcohol is effective in destroying various types of pathogens, including both viruses and bacteria, since their proteins are unfolded and inactivated. This method, called denaturation, will cripple the microbe and will sometimes kill it as its proteins will unfold and bind together.

Temperature can also denature certain proteins - the solidified egg whites are denatured proteins, for example, when you boil an egg.

2. Alcohol doesn't quite kill a few bacteria-why not?

There are various types of bacteria and viruses, and alcohol kills certain kinds with greater ease. For instance, the E. Coli bacteria, which can cause foodborne disease and other diseases, are very effectively killed at concentrations above 60 percent by alcohol.

Differences in the exterior surface of various bacteria make sanitizing alcohol more effective against some of them than others.

Similarly, some viruses have an outer covering, called an envelope, while others are unwrapped. Alcohol is effective in killing enveloped viruses, including coronavirus, but is less effective in killing germs that are not enclosed.

Whether you're trying to destroy bacteria or viruses, several scientific studies have shown that a 60 percent or higher concentration of alcohol is required to be successful.

3. When alcohol is excellent at 60 percent, is it 100 percent better?

Astonishingly, no. Denaturation of proteins generally works better when a small amount of water is combined with alcohol. And pure alcohol will evaporate too quickly to effectively destroy bacteria or viruses on your skin, mainly when the air is less humid during wintertime.

Using 100 percent alcohol will also very quickly dry out the skin and cause it to become irritated. That can cause you not to sanitize your hands as much as you need.

That's why most hand sanitizers include emollients, mixtures that help relax your skin and moisturize it.

4. Are manufactured hand sanitizers a good idea?

No, in my opinion. You can see online recipes that do-it-yourself, including those that use vodka. Yet vodka is usually 80 proof, meaning that it's only 40 percent alcohol. This is not large enough to destroy the microbes effectively.

The rubbing alcohol you have for cuts and scrapes in your bathroom might seem like a decent option, but if you're already close to a lavatory, the better choice is to wash your hands with soap and hot water.

5. Does the sanitizer hand expire?

Most commercial hand sanitizers are successful when adequately stored for a few years, and are labeled with expiry dates.

One thing to keep in mind is that alcohol is volatile, meaning the alcohol will evaporate gradually over time, and the sanitizer will lose his ability to kill viruses and bacteria efficiently. With hand sanitizer now in such high demand, though, you're unlikely to buy one that expires.

WHEN IT'S SAFE TO USE HAND SANITIZER—AND WHEN YOU NEED TO FIND SOAP AND WATER

Yeah, we remember, you were told about a bazillion times during the cold and flu season, to wash your hands daily. A brief refresher on why it's so, so important: Virus-containing droplets expelled through sneezes or coughs can be easily transmitted between people— even by merely shaking hands or grabbing a doorknob and then touching your nose or mouth.

So even in those cases, a wash with soap and water is your best option (after a flu shot, of course), a sink isn't always readily available; often you can't just pry yourself away from your office, whether you're in the midst of an outdoor workout. "You can't just be in the bathroom washing your hands all day," says Pritish K. Tosh, MD, a physician and researcher at the Mayo Clinic for infectious disease.

Join the sanitizer by hand. The alcohol-based gel plays the role of a knight in shining armor for those of us who can't help scrub-a-dub-dub around the clock from what we are doing. "It seems like an excellent idea to use them because of their simplicity and effectiveness," Dr. Tosh agrees.

And sometimes the hand sanitizer is a good idea — as long as you obey certain basic rules.

If soap and water are not available, disinfect your hands with a hand sanitizer Washing your hands with soap and water is always the first line of protection against a host of disease-inducing species, Dr. Tosh says. But when you can't get it to the sink, hand sanitizer will battle specific bugs too, like cold-causing viruses and flu.

Nonetheless, a report published in the journal Pediatrics this week poses concerns about conditions where a hand sanitizer can be more successful than washing up. The study showed that young children were less likely to get sick and skip daycare when they were using hand sanitizer than when they were washing their hands.

"Since the use of hand sanitizers is also convenient, people might be more likely to do it and use so more frequently than anyone would just stick to soap and water," Dr. Tosh hypothesizes. "And though the effectiveness [of hand sanitizer] may be smaller, there may be greater overall potential to avoid infection as it's easier to do more often." However, he says, experts aren't giving us the green light to fully skip the sink.

Should not use hand sanitizer when your hands are filthy. According to the Centers for Disease Control and Prevention (CDC), when your hands are coated in the muck, sanitizers actually will not function as well — say after you've been planting or tinkering with your bike gears.

For example, if you just apply sanitizer to the mix, the dirt and grease won't go anywhere, says TanayaBhowmick, MD, assistant professor of infectious disease medicine at the Robert Wood Johnson Medical School in New Jersey. "When you've got dirt on your hands and put alcohol on it, you're just making a slurry." She says you're going to rub the gunk around without ever washing it off.

And because hand sanitizer doesn't destroy every microbe, she underlines that there are those that you just need to wash off.

Ensure sure the sanitizer is at least 60% alcohol. The alcohol serves as what's considered a denaturing agent, explains Dr. Tosh, as opposed to soap, which serves as a detergent. Essentially, alcohol destroys or inactivates viruses— and, according to the CDC, it does so most efficiently in sanitizers that are between 60 and 95 percent alcohol.

Proper application, Dr. Bhowmick adds, is also essential. Apply hand sanitizer to one hand's palm, then "keep rubbing around all your hands until it's warm," she says. Pleasant reminder: You shouldn't have your hand sanitizer cleaned off, whether you're using a towel or your jeans ' legs (hey, we were there). "It defeats the intent, because whatever you wipe it off on, you may be picking up something else," says Dr. Bhowmick.

We like the vegan Instant Hand Sanitizer from Noodle & Boo ($10, dermstore.com), and the Advanced Hand Sanitizer from Purell with aloe ($13 for 4, amazon.com). It's a wise idea to look for an alcohol-based sanitizer with a moisturizing agent like aloe, Dr. Tosh says, because all that alcohol will dry up.

Avoid something branded as "antibacterial" If you're an obsessive user of hand sanitizer, you may have wondered if you're too full of it. Luckily, gels based on alcohol will continue to work just as well over time, so keep on rubbing on. "At least up to now, there's no evidence suggesting this isn't as successful [over time]," Dr. Bhowmick says — at least when it comes to killing viruses. Some research indicates that drug-resistant bacteria can develop an alcohol tolerance, though, she says.

That's a little worrying, considering the ever-growing danger of microbial resistance— when bacteria evolve to survive the antibiotics usually used to kill them. Dr. Tosh says that overuse of antibacterial and antimicrobial products will bolster those so-called superbugs, so stay away from the hand gels on their labels that advertise those properties.

Three Ways to Make a Natural Homemade Sanitizer

Gentle Hand Sanitizer Recipe (Safe for Kids)

A non-drying, natural hand sanitizer gel feeds on aloe vera. It's so easy to be able to help the kids make it.

Prepare Time: 1 minute

Ingredients:

- 1⁄4 cup aloe vera gel
- 20 drops destroyer germ essential oil

Combine all ingredients and store in a reusable silicone container.

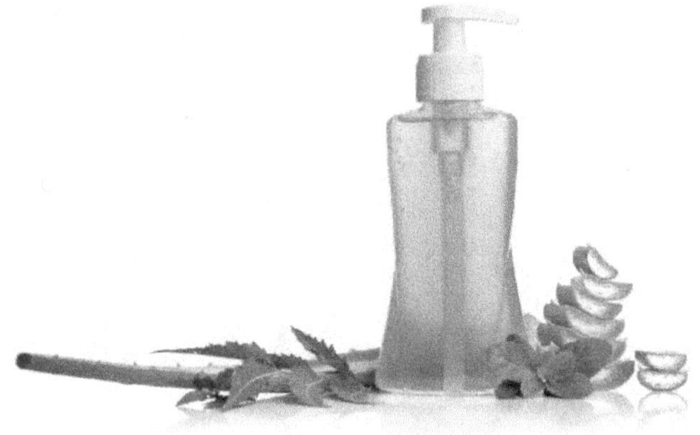

STRONGER HAND SANITIZER RECIPE

Using as needed to eliminate germs naturally from Stronger Hand Sanitizer Recipe. Use this recycle for a more reliable hand sanitizer that works like commercial versions (without the triclosan). If you're operating in a hospital, this might be a perfect one for personal use. This recycle I wouldn't use on kids!

Ingredients:

- 1 TBSP rubbing alcohol
- 1/2 tsp vegetable glycerin (optional)
- 1/4 cup aloe vera gel
- 20 drops Germ Destroyer oil
- 1 TBSP distilled water or colloidal silver / ionic silver for extra antibacterial activity
- Other essential oils (just for scent)

To produce, blend aloe vera gel, optional glycerin, and rub alcohol in a small bowl.

Add essential oil of cinnamon and tea tree oil along with a drop or two of any other oils that you wish to add for fragrance. Sweet options include lemongrass, peach, lavender, and peppermint.

Mix well and add about one tablespoon of distilled water (or ionic/colloidal silver) to thin consistency if desired.

To pass hand sanitizer into a spray or pump-style bottles, using a small funnel or medicine dropper. This can also be packed for use on the go in small silicone tubes.

Using any other form of hand sanitizer as you can.

STRONGEST HOMEMADE HAND SANITIZER RECIPE (5 MINUTE RECIPE)

To effectively kill viruses, the CDC recommends at least 60 percent alcohol in hand sanitizer. This formula follows the percentage and adds aloe vera for gentleness and essential oils for the fight against new viruses. This is the one that I'm using after working in places where the transmission of infections is more likely.

Ingredients:

- 2/3 cup alcohol rubbing (70 percent or higher)
- 2 Teaspoons aloe vera (if aloe vera can not be found, glycerin may be used as a substitute)
- 20 drops Germ Destroyer Essential Oil (You can also use Germ Fighter which is more robust, but I wouldn't recommend it for use on kids)

Mix all the ingredients and combine them in a spray bottle (these are the best size) or any small container. Use as you wish.

Keep in mind that the formula should be changed according to the strength of the alcohol you're using. For example, if you're using 99% Isopropyl rubbing alcohol, you're going to need a different amount of aloe vera than if you're using 70% alcohol. Below are some fast guidelines.

Option 1 - with 99% Isopropyl Rubbing Alcohol: two parts of alcohol and one part of aloe vera gel (e.g., 2/3 cup alcohol + 1/3 cup aloe vera gel).

Option 2 - with 91% isopropyl or rubbing alcohol: three parts whiskey and one part aloe vera gel (e.g., 3/4 cup alcohol + 1/4 cup aloe vera gel).

Option 3 - with 70% isopropyl or rubbing alcohol: nine parts of alcohol and one part of aloe vera gel.

Some people tend not to use alcohol in their hand sanitizer because alcohol has a strong odor and can have a significant drying effect on the skin.

WITCH HAZEL-BASED HAND SANITIZER

A perfect option is the use of a witch-hazel-based sanitizer. The tea tree oil has additional antiseptic benefits.

Ingredients:

- 1 cup (preferably without additives) of pure aloe vera gel
- 1/2 teaspoons hazel 30 drops tea tree oil five drops of essential oil like lavender or peppermint Spoon Funnel Glass bottle

Stir in aloe vera water, tea tree oil, and hazel witch. To thicken it, add another spoonful of aloe vera if the mixture is too thin. Remove another spoonful of witch hazel.

If it is too thick, stir the essential oil in. Since the tea tree oil's scent is already stable, the added essential oils are simple to handle. Five or so drops are meant to be enough, but mix it in one drop at a time if you want to add more.

Funn the mixture into the receptacle. Place the funnel above the jar mouth and pour in the sanitizer for the side. Fill it up, then screw it onto the lid until ready to use it.

A tiny bottle of squirt works well if you want to take the sanitizer with you all day long.

Save the remaining sanitizer in a container with a tightly fitting lid, if you make too much for the bottle.

CONCLUSION

Hand sanitizer is a convenient, on-the-gogo way to help avoid bacteria spread when there is no soap and water. Hand sanitizers based on alcohol that help to keep you healthy and reduce the spread of the novel coronavirus.

When you have trouble locating a hand sanitizer in your local stores, you should take action to make your own. Just a few ingredients are required, such as alcohol rubbing, aloe vera gel, and an essential oil or lemon juice.

While hand sanitizers can be an efficient way to get rid of germs, health officials also recommend hand washing to keep your hands clean of disease-causing viruses and other bacteria whenever possible.

DISCLAIMER

This book is not intended as a substitute for the medical advice of physicians. The reader should regularly consult a physician in matters relating to his/her health and particularly concerning any symptoms that may require diagnosis or medical attention.